Guide

John Gone

CONTENTS

1) Healthy Mind, body and Soul
2) Know what is crucial to your happiness?
3) Inspire yourself
4) Inspire and have time for other people
5) How can you make the world a better place?
6) Connecting spiritually – the death of the ego
7) Making the impossible possible – Emotional intelligence, perception
8) Be creative

ACKNOWLEDGEMENTS

I would like to dedicate this book to anybody who strives to help the well being of other people on the planet. I would also like to thank anyone who has been associated with Chipmunkapublishing and the Chipmunka Foundation over the last five years. Thank you for giving me the strength and support when I needed it most. In particular I would like to thank Andrew Latchford who is without doubt the most generous, patient and giving business partner, human being and friend that anyone could ever wish for. I would also like to thank Paul Williams, Paul Brandwood, Barbara Phillips, Mark Randall, John Bird, Nigel Kershaw, Ashley Cooke, Barbara Brown, Peter Horn, Charles Beckett, Stuart Bell, Sandra Lawman, Dominic O'Donnell, Ben Robertson, Nigel Stoneman, Rt Honourable Tony Benn, Adele Blakeborough, Robert Bond, Dolly Sen, Dominic Hiatt. Apologies if I have not mentioned you.

I would also like to thank all the Chipmunkapublishing authors for believing that they and we can make a difference. Thank you for believing in me and the Chipmunka team.

I would like to thank the many Chpimunka volunteers around the world for their time, donations, kindness and dedication in helping us to help more people. They can see that the work we are doing is a unique empowerment model that is changing the history of the mental health movement for the better.

I would like to give special thanks to the hundred and fifty or so volunteers from university students around the world who have given their time to come into Chipmunka offices to selflessly help other people whose lives need to be given a voice. I would like to give a special thanks to students from French universities and London universities for giving up a considerable amount of their time and using their initiative to help more people.

There have been many organizations and people that have helped inspire me along the way. I would like to thank Virgin, Microsoft, eBay, Apple, Manchester United, Anthony Robbins, Coldplay, Eminem, Dr Dre, Snoop Doggy Dogg, Paul McKenna, The Department of Trade & Industry, Bill Clinton,

Tony Blair, Nelson Mandela, Bob Geldof, U2, David Beckham, Madonna, Ronnie O'Sullivan, Steven Spielberg, Martin Scorsese, Ben Affleck, Matt Damon, Al Pacino, Tom Cruise, Robert de Niro, Bill Gates, Paul Merton and Richard Branson, to name but a few.

I would like to thank particular organizations that do not always get the high profile but have an important role in the well being of people in the UK especially and further a field. Please forgive me for any organizations that have not been mentioned. You know who you are. I would like to whole heartedly thank the DTI, New Statesman, The Arts Council, The National Lottery, SLAM NHS Trust, NIMHE, London Development Centre, The Sunday Times, BBC, ITV, Channel 4, Sky TV, Big Issue, Community Action Network, Mind, Rethink, Sane, the Independent, Daily Telegraph, Guardian, The Times, The Observer, Natmags, South West

News Service, Launchpad, KPMG, Faegre Benson Hobson & Audley, Olswang, mental health media, CCHR, Samaritans, NAMHE, SWNS.

I would like to thank my family and friends for allowing me to express the way I feel about the world during our time together. Thank you from the bottom of my heart. I would like to thank my partner Sonia for her love everyday that gives me the strength to continue the utopian dream that I have to eliminate the humiliation that people with 'mental health issues' feel or will ever feel and to make suicides a thing of the past. Your love, patience, kindness and advice inspire me everyday.

1   Having a healthy, mind, body and soul

To discover the ultimate path to well being, you have to reach inside of your mind, body and soul like you never have before. This takes a conscious effort or *massive action* as Anthony Robbins most aptly calls it. Anthony Robbins who is probably regarded as the greatest motivational speaker on the planet says that you need to take *massive action* in his book Unlimited Power (Published by Simon & Schuster 1989). In the last 10 years I have read several hundred self-help books and regard Unlimited Power as the best of them all, much better than his later books and audio material. He is also a pretty impressive speaker – I have listened to him for many an hour.

Anthony Robbins is exactly right. There is no point in procrastinating on doing something. You have to actually do it. You have to look inside of yourself and ask who you are as a human being and what you are capable of. Then do it.

Once you discover who you are you can then discover what you want and then start doing it. It really is as simple as that and not rocket science just life.

During this book I have decided to split the journey to Ultimate Well Being into eight manageable steps (It's like two Stephen Covey books in one – only joking, Steve I am a big fan of your books... Please keep writing). Whilst you go through each step and go through each exercise, take notes, re read anything you do not understand and visualise the positive outcomes of each step so that you are also taking a step forward and are therefore a step closer to Ultimate Well Being. Each step will take you that little bit closer to 100% mental well being. See this book as an examination of yourself. You will be able to pass but you will have to challenge yourself to progress. This book is an opportunity for you to test yourself and give yourself 100% success as you are the examiner of your life. Nobody else is responsible for how you feel… Just you… That is the reality. See this examination as a confirmation that you and anyone can choose to be a success and even rid yourself of your ego in the process so you can lead a more fulfilled life and have a more positive impact on the world. I repeat. You are the examiner in your life. Ultimately no matter where you seek inspiration the responsibility of living your life boils down to you and not anybody else.

This is not just another self help book. Even if it was I do not think that would necessarily be a bad thing. I like self help books. They fill your head with positive things and day to day people can easily be bombarded with more negative than positive thoughts so a self-help can reprogramme positivism. My first two books document how I lived a life of manic depression and cured myself. (If you feel this is dubious please break your pattern, open your mind, change your belief system do whatever it takes to accept this as fact and then read on!) I have been in the depths of despair and welcomed positivism and enlightenment into my life and made the permanent switch into having a happy mind, body and soul. Therefore I am qualified to write a new type of self-help book and publish a new type of self-help genre of autobiographical memoirs from people who suffer 'mental illness' as I have changed my life and I am not using some kind of theoretical system like most other self help books where the personal suffering or the author and their biographical/autobiographical history and weaknesses are a mystery. Reading this book is a unique opportunity for you to totally enhance your life and reach new standards in every aspect of your life so you can be totally empowered.

You will be able to be a *novus homo* as they say in Latin. A new man as the amazing Roman orator Cicero was in 63BC when he became a member of the Equestrian Order through his achievements instead of through birth. Nobody had done that previously in the history of Rome so it really was an outstanding achievement. If you find it hard to identify with the life of someone over 2000 years ago in another city then think of rap.

Think of Eminem's lyrics in the film 8 Mile. The Director of 8 Mile said that writing the lyrics for 8 Mile made Eminem go deeper inside himself than at any other time in his life. As Eminem says in the most famous track he wrote for the movie "*If you had one chance, one opportunity in life… would you capture it or let it slip*". The implication is that you capture it and this is exactly what Eminem does in the film 8 Mile and exactly why he won the contest and went back to work to save up for his studio time so Rabbit would become a famous rapper just like Eminem is.

Would you capture it or let it slip?

I remember being inspired when watching 8 Mile and was fortunate that when an opportunity came along for me to make a rap album I managed to capture it and not let it slip. I have recently launched this rap album. Although it was a very steep learning curve over a short period of time and a lot of hard work it was much easier than I thought. The album is called "A Can of Madness", the same name of my book and autobiography on living with manic depression published in 2002 by Chipmunkapublishing. I had once chance to do a rap album and took it. It all started when a volunteer in the Chipmunka office called Ama was reading the rap I wrote in "A Can of Madness" and said that she liked it and that she had a friend whose boyfriend was a rapper. I've always loved hip-hop ever since I heard NWA's 'Straight Outta Compton' at the age of 12. I see hip-hop as a potential force for good to bring cultures together and stop racism globally. I liked writing lyrics but never really thought of doing an album or performing. Soon enough I met Ama's friend and the rapper. His name was Ryan and at 17 years of age he had his own label Raskil Records. I was amazed how good the rappers were on his label, especially as most of them were teenagers and they wanted to help people with mental illness so within 6 weeks I had paid for and organised two rap events for them to perform for the very first time live. At the first event one of my friends came along whose rap name is Howling. He was 23 years of age at the time and multi-talented and introduced me to his friend Avarice who made his beats. Avarice happens to be a brilliant producer, lyricist and rapper himself and went out of his way to help. We held several sessions after work in my office and Avarice had given me a crash course in rapping in time to the beats to the lyrics that I had written a few years earlier. This consisted of several evening sessions after work in Chipmunka's main offices in central London. Then we spent one day round his house as he has his own studio and within four months of meeting him I had launched my rap album.

    I mention this as an example to you that not only like Eminem you can do anything like making a rap album if you wanted to. It's just a little example of how if you have a good feeling for something that you should just go for it and reap the rewards whether they are emotional, financial, psychological or spiritual. In return I wanted to help Avarice so kept in touch and I am helping to promote his crew Renegade Artistry. Check them out at www.rarecords.net. They really are some of the most talented rappers in British Hip Hop.

Moment of Decision

As Anthony Robbins tells us it is in the moment of our decision when our lives change or make a *paradigm shift* as Stephen Covey calls it. Anyone who hears and connects with Eminem in the film 8 Mile could think of something in their lives that they have been hesitant about and would choose to go for it. If you read this book with this positive mentality and decisiveness then you will achieve Ultimate Well Being.

So congratulations to you dear reader for taking that quantum leap (Yes VISUALISE IT RIGHT NOW... feel good... that's not good enough.... feel great... feel fantastic... that's more like it!!!) into a happier state of consciousness... OK... THEN LET'S PROCEED...

We get what we focus on in life. In order to have a healthy mind, body and soul you need to treat these conditions as achievable qualities. Everyone has them so if you don't feel it stop moping around and just zap yourself with some amazing, fantastic, energising sense of feeling great for yourself, other people and the world as a whole. If someone tells you that you have manic depression and a chemical imbalance in the brain, they do not know what they are talking about. You can alter your chemistry by getting more oxygen and jogging in the morning. No psychiatrist has ever proven that there is something wrong with your brain so snap out of believing it. Life is worth living. Take it from me I know I have been so low I was suicidal for months at a time and I chose life just like Renton did in Trainspotting. If you haven't seen that movie go and watch it and then watch the last 5 minutes again. feel the sensation of turning your life around. It really is that is easy. If Forest Gump can achieve the impossible then so can you my dear friend. And if you can… so can anyone…

So let's deconstruct having a healthy mind, body and soul into three parts. First let's break them down into three separate parts. Then we will show how they are all connected.

Having a healthy mind.

Having a healthy mind is as achievable as you want it to be. Let's set some targets. Say out loud "my goal is to have a healthy mind body and soul 24 hours a day seven days a week for the rest of my life." Feel good? Well good isn't good enough…. feel very good…. feel outstanding……. Woooooooooooowwwwhhhhhh…… Great. Say it again first in your mind. Then out loud. Now try doing something fun with your body, like smiling, while you are doing this or even be more adventurous and try a flying kick... something to give you more oxygen and change your physiology so you are in a PEAK state....... Repeat this three times... Feeling Great..... Now CONTINUE.

Those of you who have been to an Anthony Robbins Seminar will know exactly what I am talking about. Don't worry if you haven't. Ever seen Paul McKenna? Now you have re-programmed your mind as Paul McKenna would say to make this feeling of feeling GREAT a reality. The more intensely you practice this INCANTATION and awaken the more real it will become. Why not commit to chanting to your first step to Ultimate Well Being three times a day for the next year, after that it will be automatic. Now you have programmed your mind to choose a healthy mind you can mark yourself and give yourself 1% towards Ultimate Well Being.

Congratulations, you only have 99% to go. This will be as

easy as you wish it to be. And you will remember the decisions you have made in this book forever because you are consciously choosing to do so. Now celebrate as if your favourite football team has just scored! Or for all you ladies reading this as if you have just bought a beautiful outfit that you feel stunning in and the man or woman of your dreams walks straight up to you and asks you out. LOL... Or something else that will give you the same amazing feeling. Having just met your loved one for the first time! An end to world poverty... Every religion becoming friends... Something totally awesome and loving so you will NEVER FORGET THIS BEAUTIFUL MOMENT. Do whatever it takes to make this crucial moment in your personal development last forever and then multiply the love and intensity a MILLION TIMES. Close your eyes and have some beautiful intensity and love that will improve your life and the lives of those you love and even those that you haven't met forever. Feel the love and relax in a state of being.

Congratulations you are now fully on your way to ACHIEVING 100% and ULTIMATE WELL BEING, What's remarkable too is that this is a gift that you can pass on both consciously and unconsciously. You can pass this on so you can help other people and the world as one. Eckhart Tolle writes about this in The Power of Now. He is an amazing person. For the first 29 years of his life he was severely mentally ill. Then a profound spiritual transformation virtually dissolved his old identity and radically changed the course of his life. He did not know who he was but spent three years on a spiritual high and lived for two years on a park bench in a state of ecstasy. The transition that transformed his life happened in a split second. Eckhart Tolle writes in his introduction of the Power of Now that he lived in a state of almost continuous anxiety interspersed with periods of suicidal depression. One night he woke up with absolute dread that was so intense, more intense than he had ever experienced. He had a deep loathing for everything in the world his misery was compounded as he loathed himself more than anything else. During his moment of the deepest psychological pain that he ever experienced he broke through in to a higher state of consciousness. Tolle writes:

"I cannot live with myself any longer." This was the thought that kept repeating itself in my mind. Then suddenly I became aware of what a peculiar thought it was. "Am I one or two? If I cannot live with myself, there must be two of me: the 'I' and the 'self' that 'I' cannot live with. "Maybe," I thought, "only one of them is real."

His massive action, paradigm step, step into Ultimate Well Being, step into being, personal transformation or whatever you want to call it, shows that anything is possible for a human being. Tolle is a living example that anyone's life no matter how desperate can improve.

The same is true of any kind of mental illness including manic depression. I know this because I achieved the transition myself. When I was 17 I was diagnosed with manic depression. From the ages 17-25 I spent over 1 year of my life in five different psychiatric hospitals. By the age of 29 I had made a 90% recovery but was still part of the medical system. In September 2005 I made a life changing decision after meeting Robbins who work I'd been following and using as one of my techniques for inspiration in life and work for five years to take the final step to constant empowerment and Ultimate Well Being by accepting that my manic depression was entirely self manifested and that I would come off the medication that was poisoning my mind and to come off it forever. I also managed to get sponsored by the NHS to go to his events so that was a bonus and felt justified in receiving this gift as my day job is a social entrepreneur and learning his techniques would enable me to help more people anyway. Robbins and his techniques had helped but without being a social entrepreneur I would never had been able to make a full recovery. Both positive outcomes could be maximised to help even more people and give myself more personal growth and happiness.

    Within four months of attending Robbins with 12,000 other people hugging each other four for days which was an uplifting experience that I will always cherish I'd come off medication for good and had 25 people working for me full-time for free at my company Chipmunkapublishing's first offices in London. This accelerated the utopian vision to change the way the world thinks about mental health and facilitated the launch of the Chipmunka Foundation

(Registered charity number 1109537) and enabled me to help more people worldwide.

Every second of every day I looked inside my inner self, looking at what was truly important to me as a human being. As my mind became free of medication I became stronger every day and more fun to be around.

Within eight months of deciding to come off my life had totally changed. I spent three months coming off slowly with discussions with my psychiatrist who could see that I had massive insight into my own behaviour, life and belief systems and he gave me his full consent and support because he could see that I had total commitment with the intelligence, aptitude and mental strength to make a life changing commitment forever.

Now my psychiatrist is an active supporter in the active goals of my social enterprises and charity. How great is that? If you are a psychiatric patient this shows that you can totally cure yourself not just philosophically but in reality. It is just as easy as choosing to and following up whatever you want to do in life.

By May 2005 I was sat in a room with 200 people at the Dali museum in London listening to the Channel 4 TV presenter Sarah Smith talking about how I had a vision for the world which shows massive potential for helping people cure themselves of mental illness, I was a phenomenal public speaker, extremely talented, consultant, social entrepreneur who had written one of the most defining books of his generation etc... A few seconds later I was awarded the New Statesman's Young Social Entrepreneur of the year 2005, beating celebrity chef Jamie Oliver who has in own TV series and had convinced Tony Blair to commit to spending more money on every school dinner for pupils in schools throughout the country. All my dreams were starting to come true at a quicker pace because I had been setting the appropriate plans but also because I had chosen to take massive action myself and actually do it. I'd decided that it was only me who was responsible for what happened in my life. This is true for you too. If you want a healthy mind, body, soul or anything else in life then ultimately it is your responsibility to do something about it.

    Now repeat after me: Me, myself and I choose to achieve 100% mental well being and I choose to do so now. Feel it, visualise it, imagine it, celebrate it.... do it... Happy.... Feeling great.... Play your favourite song, shout it out, do it with a friend, meditate, play football or do martial arts while you are saying this to get more oxygen in your body... Do whatever it takes to make it have a stronger and more lasting impact on your new found content and happy mind. Do this with your friend, partner, imaginary friend, remote control or any other inanimate object next to this book. Do it now, enjoy it and celebrate as if you have just won your favourite Olympic event and then donated your gold medal to charity for world peace… and say it five times so it stays with you.

Say that you will do it five times for the next five days and it will stay with you. Then every five days it becomes five times more intense and five times the fun. Who would not want that great felling to continue? Congratulations you can now give yourself 2% in your journey to 100% mental well being and Ultimate Well Being.

Just like anyone else who is a PEAK PERFORMER I constantly draw inspiration from people who have the greatest minds in history to challenge me everyday in my own mind and life so that I can help the people that The Chipmunka Group is designed to help. Some of my favourite inspirational figures in this world are:

1) Mohandas Gandhi (1869-1948). Known as Mahatma

('Great-Soul'), Gandhi was the leader of the Indian nationalist movement against British rule, and is widely considered the father of his country. His doctrine of non-violent protest to achieve political and social progress has been hugely influential.

Gandhi stuck to what he believed in. He had the peace of mind to continue non violent and peaceful demonstrations despite being constantly pushed to the edge where most people have cracked under pressure and changed strategies even beginning to use violence. Gandhi stuck to his principles, made a bigger impact than using force would have done and went down in history as a force for social greatness.

2) From 1931 to 1948 Mother Teresa taught at St. Mary's High School in Calcutta, but the suffering and poverty she glimpsed outside the convent

walls made such a deep impression on her that in 1948 she received permission from her superiors to leave the convent school and devote herself to working among the poorest of the poor in the slums of Calcutta. Although she had no funds, she depended on Divine Providence, and started an open-air school for slum children. Soon she was joined by voluntary helpers, and financial support was also forthcoming. This made it possible for her to extend the scope of her work.

On October 7, 1950, Mother Teresa received permission from the Holy See to start her own order, "The Missionaries of Charity", whose primary task was to love and care for those persons nobody was prepared to look after. In 1965 the Society became an

International Religious Family by a decree of Pope Paul VI.

The Society of Missionaries has spread all over the world, including the former Soviet Union and Eastern European countries. They provide effective help to the poorest of the poor in a number of countries in Asia, Africa, and Latin America, and they undertake relief work in the wake of natural catastrophes such as floods, epidemics, and famine, and for refugees. The order also has houses in North America, Europe and Australia, where they take care of the shut-ins, alcoholics, homeless, and AIDS sufferers. Mother Teresa is also someone whose mind I admire. She dedicated her life to helping other people less fortunate than herself. She goes down as number two in my list of most inspirational minds in my mind today.

3) I am also greatly inspired as many people are by the mind of Nelson Mandela. Nelson Mandela is one of the world's most revered statesman, who led the struggle to replace the apartheid regime of South Africa with a multi-racial democracy.

Despite many years in jail, he emerged to become the country's first black president and to play a leading role in the drive for peace in other spheres of conflict. He won the Nobel Peace Prize in 1993.

Bob Geldof was right to call him the president of the world. Nelson Mandela gave his life to stop the suffering and discrimination felt by his people. He reaches my top ten minds today. My top minds may change on a daily basis as yours can as there thousands of people that inspire me to push myself further and enable me to lead a more fulfilled, meaningful and loving life.

4) John Lennon also had an amazing mind. John Lennon's mind is so creative and he has given joy to millions of people. He created his own music and the Beatles are the most successful band in history. I like the way John Lennon went through stages and experimented with his mind. From songs such as Jealous Guy, All You Need is Love, his boyish humour and his peace demonstrations. His mind and his actions are truly inspirational to me.

5) Like many other people I have respect for Albert Einstein. Einstein changed the way we all think about by his theory of Relativity! I was never very good at Science at school but like many other people I am inspired by Einstein's positive impact on the world. Einstein contributed more than any other scientist to the modern vision of physical reality. His special and general

theories of relativity are still regarded as the most satisfactory model of the large-scale universe that we have.

(6) Pele was a genius on the football pitch. Pele was the greatest footballer of all time in many people's books, scoring over 1000 goals in his career. He stormed on the scene in the 1970 World Cup. He had a quick mind for football. He applied his mind to a higher standard than others and was an amazing player to watch. By 1970 people thought that he was past it but he led Brazil to winning the world cup that year and was inspirational in the tournament. I am a big sports fan and watching the greats like Pele is one reason why I still enjoy playing football. I could quite easily come up with a list of 10 sportsmen who inspire me on a daily basis.

(7) I have always loved playing chess. Gary Kasparov makes my top ten minds of all time for today as he is probably the greatest

chess player of all time. I know how demanding chess is mentally and physically as I played to a high competitive standard from the age of seven. Kasparov has won world titles and dominated the game for well over a decade. Kasparov is also an amazing person as he speaks articulately on human rights issues.

(8) Marcus Tallies Cicero, the famous Roman orator was the statesman, humanitarian and lawyer who was born 106BC-died 43BC is one of my heroes of history. He rose from plebeian to statesman class which was unprecedented and chose not to become a dictator in 60BC when asked to join the First Triumvirate as he was not corrupted by political power. His philosophical work On Old Age is also the most sensible and helpful philosophical essay that I have ever written. It actually makes you look forward to Old Age.

9) Other minds that inspire me include William Shakespeare.

Shakespeare wrote many amazing plays and beautiful sonnets which are still played and known to people all over the world of all ages nearly 400 years after his death. His plays and poems move people through every single emotion: joy fear, sorrow, pain, pleasure, humour, despair and enlightenment. Shakespeare's work touches every single facet of human emotion and has stood the test of time.

10) I also have a great deal of respect for Thomas Ssazz who has challenged psychiatry since the 1960s. Ssazz's writing has pioneered much service user thinking about psychiatry today and shown that the drug companies grip on the world of mental health patients worldwide need not last forever and can convince people to think in different ways.

    I constantly use people throughout history to inspire me so I have a mindset that keeps me on my toes and raises my standards every second of every day. You can do the same. Write down the ten greatest minds that inspire you. Think of people who have changed the world or people who have had a profound impact on history, politics, sport, art, literature. Even if it is your friends or family that inspire you most write their names down and then give reasons why.

Your top 10 minds

1
2
3
4
5
6
7
8
9
10

Finished your list now? That's great. You have now achieved 3% of your Ultimate Well Being. Write a line or two for each explaining how they inspire you to increase your score to 4%

1

2

3

4

5

6

7

8

9

10

_____
_____
_____

Now you have finished your list of people that inspire you and the reasons how they inspire read each person's name and the reasons out loud with passion in the same way you read out your incantation. Congratulations you have now achieved 5% mental well being. Feeling good… ok…. FEELING GREAT……… that's better. I deliberately made the first few steps the most difficult.

Now achieving your well being score should become easier as you go through the exercises.

NLP

The mind as you can see is an extremely powerful tool and so is the body. People who study NLP (Neuron-Linguistic Programming) realize now how important the way we use our bodies is. Fifty-five percent of how we communicate is through our physiology. Only 7% is from the words we use and 38% is from sound and tonality of the way we do things. Imagine you walk around standing upright, walking confidently and with an expression of calmness and friendliness. You will be able to send a positive vibe or give positive chi when you come into contact with people, if you maintain this positivism. You can even go further and deliberately be nice to people. This will have a positive impact on their day and yours. This is much better than walking and dragging your feet kicking, cussing, being cynical and placing your problems on other people etc… better stop there. I do not want to break your pattern and make you sad. Let's keep it up and positive. Happy… move on… Just a word of warning for you, don't be overly nice to people on an ongoing basis as this is not being honest with people. Better to be positive than negative though, as this is really important in your journey to Ultimate Well Being.

Think about the following. If you see someone walking down the road, looking angry, cursing and swearing, this will put your body in a different state… Your physiology will drop in somehow… turn negative… Your heart rate may increase… you may remember something that annoys you and your mood will drop as well… You may even cross the road… You may change the way you breathe or stop breathing… This could make you nervous… stressed… anxious…. give you a panic attack.... even give you Conversion Syndrome Disorder if you repeated this behaviour over a number of years...

See how the previous mindset triggered and caused this negativity.... It was self manifested.... You could do the exact opposite.... Think about it. You've already mastered your mind. You have the 10 greatest minds in history inspiring you and you know you can visualize more amazing people inspiring you in any walk of life at any moment to help you get to achieve whatever you want to in life......you can move forward at any moment when using your mind. You can do the same with your body too....

Walk down the road.... smile... look at someone else and feel happy and smile... Your positive chi will pass onto the next person and so on... You will walk confidently... your physiology will be strong.... You will enjoy every second.... look forward to what you are going to do and be happy in that present moment… and have a great day... This is something you chose and something that you decided to do.

I am now 31 years of age and my body is in better shape than it has ever been. I have more energy than I have ever had and average 6.30 hours sleep a day because that is all I require to have an amazing day each day. I believe that I am lucky to have a healthy body and look after it by eating healthy, exercising daily and not smoking. I believe that the healthier my body, the healthier and happier I am as a human being.

I know the positive impacts of a healthy lifestyle and playing football and or exercising most days, releases positive endorphins in my body that make me physically and therefore psychologically happier than I would have been without exercising.

I still admire people in history who have the healthiest bodies of all time and step into their shoes to give me a psychological buzz at every opportunity I have consciously and unconsciously chosen to improve the condition of my body, which I know helps my related state, emotional well being and happiness.

Inspirational Bodies

(1) I have an amazing amount of respect for Lance Armstrong. Lance Armstrong won the Tour De France 6 times. The Tour De France is one of the most demanding physical challenges in any sporting event. No-one else has won the Tour as many times as Lance Armstrong or as many times in a row. What makes the life of Lance Armstrong even more incredible is that he became ill with cancer, nearly died and still came back to win the Tour De France on his return. You think he did this by feeling sorry for himself... no way... he

achieved this by deciding that he could overcome it and kept that positive mindset throughout.

(2) Second on my list of bodies that inspire me is Arnold Schwarzenegger. Arnold Schwarzenegger was born in a small town in Austria and became Mr. Universe 5 times. He trained unbelievably hard. When I used to play competitive rugby as a teenager it was Arnold Schwarzenegger who inspired me to go down to the gym even though I had never met him. I knew no matter how many times I went to the gym that Arnold Schwarzenegger would look stronger than me. Imagining him as a potential opponent and imagining I was him when training inspired me to train more frequently and train harder. Rugby, like many sports is quite a psychological game and the stronger you look to your opponent and the stronger you feel and are makes a difference.

(3) Third in my list of remarkable bodies is Bruce Lee. He was renowned as the greatest martial artist in the world and was responsible for taking martial arts into Hollywood. In 1970 (Age 30): Bruce had injured his sacral nerve and experiences severe muscle spasms in his back while training. Doctors told him that he would never kick again. During the months of recovery he starts to document his training methods and his philosophy of Jeet Kune Do. Thirty years later this martial art is revered and practised all over the world and Bruce Lee inspires thousands of people to take up martial arts every year.

(4) Another body or person that I admire is Amir Khan. At 17 years of age he went to the Olympics and gained a sliver medal. Less than a year later he turned professional and beat the boxer who beat him in the final, has won his first ten professional fights and looks set to become a future World Boxing Champion.

(5) Houdini is the most famous magician of all time. Houdini is credited with the invention or unique improvement of a number of important illusions (the Strait Jacket Escape, Walking Through a Brick Wall, Metamorphosis, Buried Alive, the Hindu Needle Trick, the Chinese Water Torture Cell and the Milk Can Escape). He revolutionized magic and took it to another level. He could escape from things that other people could never have perceived before.

6) The most amazing magician and stunt performer David Blaine is also somebody who inspires me. David Blaine (4/04/1973 from Brooklyn, New York City) made his name as a performer of street and close-up magic. David Blaine has performed many stunts. For example in November 2000 Blaine began a stunt called "Frozen In Time". Blaine stood in a closet of ice which was sculpted to fit his body, and a tube provided him with air and

water while his urine was removed from another tube. He was encased in ice for 61 hours, 40 minutes and 15 seconds before being removed. Blaine survived as the whole world witnessed the event on television.

(7) I remember when I was 9 years old watching the Los Angeles Olympics on Television. Carl Lewis won the 100 metres, 200 metres, long jump and relay. On the biggest day of his life he succeeded and was at the top of his sport for several years. All together he won 9 Olympic gold medals and 8 world championship gold medals. Although I never went on to enter the Olympics I found Carl Lewis an inspirational figure during and after that Olympics.

(8) Steven Redgrave is another amazing athlete. He is the only athlete in the history of the Olympics to win a gold medal in 5 different Olympics. Redgrave epitomizes the success that an individual can have at peak

performance for the longest interval. He has also won the BBC's sports personality of the year.

9) Phil Taylor is someone who deserves a lot of admiration. He has fantastic eye sight and hand to eye coordination. Phil Taylor was born on 13/08/60 and is a multi word champion darts player, considered by most to be the greatest ever. His nickname is 'The Power'. Taylor has now clocked up 11 PDC World Championships to bring his haul to 13 world titles. Knowing how hard he practices I would not bet against him winning any more world titles.

10) Michael Jordan is another amazing athlete. He is the greatest basketball player of all time. He also made a comeback at the age of 35. Jordan put in the effort. He practiced before everyone else did for 1 year when his high school coach refused to pick him. Next year he

got in the team and the rest is history.

Now think of 10 people with the most amazing bodies in history that inspire you.

1
2
3
4
5
6
7
8
9
10

Great……. Well Done…. Feel the rush….. Feel the buzz…… Coming up…. GETTING HIGHER. Feel that natural feeling of Ultimate Well Being….

Now you are 6% on your way to Ultimate Well Being. Write a line or two on why each one inspires you to get to 7%.

1

2

3

4

5

6

7

8

9

10

Read out loudly the names of the people whose bodies inspire you and why and you have 8% Ultimate Well Being. Congratulations. You are well on your way to leading a happier life....

Having a healthy Soul

Make sure you do not mention the same people in this section as you did in the healthy mind or body section. That would make it too easy.... Draw inspiration from different sources to maximize your well being.

Now you have a healthy mind and body why not go all the way and choose to have a healthy soul. There are many people throughout history who have a healthy soul.

(1) Top of my list today is Jesus. I was born a Christian but I am not particularly religious. I see myself more as a humanitarian with a mindset similar to some aspects of Buddhism. Like many people I see myself as someone who draws inspiration from everyone who has a positive impact on the world. I see my duty in life as a

communicator of Ultimate Well Being and Mental Health Empowerment. Whatever your religious beliefs Jesus was an amazingly generous person. Two thousand years after he walked the earth, Jesus of Nazareth remains one of those most talked-about and influential people who has ever lived. Jesus dedicated his life to helping others and even died for us. How's that for having a beautiful soul.

(2) Martin Luther King also had an amazing soul. He was instrumental in giving black people a voice in America, reducing racism and giving equality to black people throughout the world. He died for what he believed in and has had a positive impact on the whole world.

(3) In my mind, Bill Gates has an amazing soul. He had a dream to give everyone in the world the opportunity to have their own computer. He has been the

richest man in the world for the last decade but gives away a high percentage of his wealth for charitable causes.

(4) Dale Carnegie also has a beautiful soul. He was the wealthiest man in the world and was ruthless but then went back to a commitment that he made at the age of 30. By the time he would die, he promised to redistribute his wealth for the benefit of society and for the education of the world and he made sure he did. He accomplished so much, setting up schools and libraries that would not have been set up without his help.

(5) In my view Anthony Robbins, the world's leader in motivational seminars, also has a beautiful soul. He is driven by the will to encourage everyone he meets to reach their full potential in life.

Now come up with 5 souls in the world that you inspire. It can be famous people or people you know.

1
2
3
4
5

You know the score... Twenty Thousand hardcore knocking at your door... Only joking... Write a line or two on why each of them inspires you to take your well being score to 10%. Celebrate.... Jump up in the air... SMILE TO YOURSELF... however you want. Enjoy the natural rush and feeling of Ultimate Well Being.

1

2

3

4

5

When you have written this down and read it out loud and agree to at the utmost intensity like you have never meant anything before, you will have completed 11% of your journey to Ultimate Well Being.

As you have gone through each exercise, you may have been thinking of the same people for different categories. I know I did. I asked you not to repeat the same people to make your journey to ultimate well being more rewarding and more soul searching. I never said it was going to be easy but I promise you if you follow the techniques in this book verbatim and give everything that you've got, then you will be able to move forward and have the opportunity to make 100% ultimate well being a reality. There is no reason why you will not be able to keep that reality. This choice has already been made by you so congratulations once again.... you are well on your way to Ultimate Well Being.

You will see now that there are people who can fit into all these categories and people who do not for one reason or other. To achieve 100% mental well being you have to succeed in every category. Winston Churchill had a great mind. He was Prime minister, he had a great soul, he is said to have saved Britain in its hour of need. He didn't need much sleep. He was overweight, a drunk and a smoker and suffered from depression. In my eyes Churchill fails in one category, possibly two so realize how far you are going to stretch yourself. You are now only at 11% so there is a long way to go but you can choose to do it. Be like NIKE or somebody who inspires you- Just do it.

You can go further in your guide to Ultimate Well Being than Winston Churchill did, one of the most accomplished statesmen of the 20th Century. There is no reason why you can't be successful in all three categories. I have a healthy mind, body and soul because I have identified what constitutes having a healthy mind, body soul every day means for me.

When I worked out what having a healthy mind means to me I decided that it meant a mind free from medication, drugs and alcohol abuse. I choose to use my mind everyday to spend time doing what I am passionate about and learning more and more about philanthropy, social entrepreneurship, mental health, well being, business practices social justice, information technology, Neuron-Linguistic Programming, the world and other things. I learnt to appreciate my friends and family more and appreciate simple things in life and the now and not worry so much about the past and the future.

I see life as a gift and I believe that I have an opportunity and duty to use the previous pain that I have experienced as a former manic depressive as a force for social good to have a positive impact on the world. I believe that I can facilitate changing the way the world thinks about mental health for the better and empower millions of people around the world to empower each other and give each other a voice so that in 50 years time there will be no humiliation for anyone who is regarded as "mentally ill". The moment that I realized I was in a mental institution at the age of 17, was the defining moment of my life. The first thought that went through my mind was that the humiliation I felt was unjust and I knew that when I chose to, I would spend the rest of my life finding a way to prevent other people going through the same humiliation that I felt.

I can say three things about having a healthy mind, body and soul.

1 My healthy mind is a crucial tool in reaching the most important personal goals in my life.

www.ingramcontent.com/pod-product-compliance
Lightning Source LLC
Chambersburg PA
CBHW020810160426
43192CB00006B/517